I would like to dedicate this book to my parents,
Babu and Nadasha,
my sister Sibina and my beloved Kuttoose
Without their encouragement
it wasn't possible for me to write this book.

I also dedicate it to my wonderful and supportive masters,

Shifu Vineesh.R.P

Shihan P.S.Unnikrishnan

E.S.Narayanan Gurukkal

CONTENTS

INTRODUCTION

Overweight and obesity are defined as "abnormal or excessive fat accumulation that presents a risk to health". Being overweight is especially common where food supplies are plentiful and lifestyles are sedentary.   As of 2003, excess weight reached epidemic proportions globally, with more than 1 billion adults being either overweight or obese. In 2013 this increased to more than 2 billion Increases have been observed across all age groups. A healthy body requires a minimum amount of fat for proper functioning of the hormonal, reproductive, and immune systems, as thermal insulation, as shock absorption for sensitive areas, and as energy for future use. But the accumulation of too much storage fat can impair movement, flexibility, and alter the appearance of the body.

The degree to which a person is overweight is generally described by the body mass index (BMI). *Overweight* is defined as a BMI of 25 or more, thus it includes pre-obesity defined as a BMI between 25 and 30 and obesity as defined by a BMI of 30 or more. Pre-obese and overweight however are often used interchangeably, thus giving overweight a common definition of a BMI of between 25–30. There are, however, several other common ways to measure the amount of adiposity or fat present in an individual's body.

There are many factors that may contribute to this imbalance include:

>   Alcoholism.
>   Eating disorders (such as binge eating).
>   Genetic predisposition.
>   Hormonal imbalances (e.g. hypothyroidism).
>   Insufficient or poor-quality sleep.
>   Limited physical exercise and a sedentary lifestyle.
>   Poor nutrition.

> Metabolic disorders, which could be caused by repeated attempts to lose weight by weight cycling.
> Overeating.
> Psychotropic medication (e.g. olanzapine).
> Smoking cessation and other stimulant withdrawal.
> Stress.

Overweight and obesity may increase the risk of many health problems, including diabetes, heart disease, and certain cancers. If you are pregnant, excess weight may lead to short- and long-term health problems for you and your child. Excess weight may increase the risk for many health problems, including :

> Type 2 diabetes.
> High blood pressure.
> Heart disease and strokes.
> Certain types of cancer.
> sSeep apnea.
> Osteoarthritis.
> Fatty liver disease.
> Kidney disease.
> Pregnancy problems, such as high blood sugar during pregnancy, high blood pressure, and increased risk for cesarean delivery (C-section).

Doing yoga regularly offers many benefits, including making you feel better about your body as you become stronger and more flexible, toning your muscles, reducing stress, and improving your mental and physical well-being. But how can it help you lose weight? Practicing any type of yoga will build strength, In order to lose weight, you must eat healthily and burn calories by doing exercise that raises your heart rate on a regular basis. More vigorous yoga styles can provide a better workout than gentle yoga. Yoga can play an important role in a weight loss program.While losing weight can be simplified to a calories in vs. calories out equation, a lot more goes into successfully changing your habits to make healthier choices second nature. Yoga helps by bringing you better in tune with your body, improving your self-image and sense of well-being. Reducing stress and thereby stress eating is another way that yoga can support weight loss. By encouraging a healthy lifestyle, consistent yoga practice makes it more likely that you'll be able to maintain your weight loss. Perhaps most significantly, yoga's emphasis on listening to your body first and foremost can be a sea change for people who have struggled to shed pounds in the past. Yoga has an important role to play in a holistic approach to weight loss.In this book I provide you a unique yogic system that combines all aspects of yoga includes yogasanas, Pranayama, Mudras, and Meditation.With the help of this book you can lose weight in 21 days.Al you have to do is follow the instructions for 21 days .Patience and practice is the key to success.

1

OVERWEIGHT AND OBESITY MEASURES

It is difficult to develop one simple index for the measurement of overweight and obesity in children and adolescents because their bodies undergo a number of physiological changes as they grow. Depending on the age, different methods to measure a body's healthy weight are available:

How can you tell if your weight could increase your chances of developing health problems? Knowing two numbers may help you understand your risk: your **Body mass index (BMI)** score and your **waist size** in inches.

Body Mass Index

The BMI is one way to tell whether you are at a normal weight, are overweight, or have obesity. It measures your weight in relation to your height and provides a score to help place you in a category:

➢ Normal weight: BMI of 18.5 to 24.9
➢ Overweight: BMI of 25 to 29.9
➢ Obesity: BMI of 30 or higher

Charts and tables, such as the one below, are one easy way to figure out your BMI. There are also several online BMI calculators To use the table below, find your height on the left side of the chart, then go across to the weight that is closest to yours. At the top of the chart you can see your BMI, and at the bottom of the chart you can see which category you fit into – healthy weight, overweight, or obese:

TABLE 2   Adult BMI Chart

BMI	19	20	21	22	23	24	25	26	27	28	29	30	31	32	33	34	35
Height							Weight in Pounds										
4'10"	91	96	100	105	110	115	119	124	129	134	138	143	148	153	158	162	167
4'11"	94	99	104	109	114	119	124	128	133	138	143	148	153	158	163	168	173
5'	97	102	107	112	118	123	128	133	138	143	148	153	158	163	168	174	179
5'1"	100	106	111	116	122	127	132	137	143	148	153	158	164	169	174	180	185
5'2"	104	109	115	120	126	131	136	142	147	153	158	164	169	175	180	186	191
5'3"	107	113	118	124	130	135	141	146	152	158	163	169	175	180	186	191	197
5'4"	110	116	122	128	134	140	145	151	157	163	169	174	180	186	192	197	204
5'5"	114	120	126	132	138	144	150	156	162	168	174	180	186	192	198	204	210
5'6"	118	124	130	136	142	148	155	161	167	173	179	186	192	198	204	210	216
5'7"	121	127	134	140	146	153	159	166	172	178	185	191	198	204	211	217	223
5'8"	125	131	138	144	151	158	164	171	177	184	190	197	203	210	216	223	230
5'9"	128	135	142	149	155	162	169	176	182	189	196	203	209	216	223	230	236
5'10"	132	139	146	153	160	167	174	181	188	195	202	209	216	222	229	236	243
5'11"	136	143	150	157	165	172	179	186	193	200	208	215	222	229	236	243	250
6'	140	147	154	162	169	177	184	191	199	206	213	221	228	235	242	250	258
6'1"	144	151	159	166	174	182	189	197	204	212	219	227	235	242	250	257	265
6'2"	148	155	163	171	179	186	194	202	210	218	225	233	241	249	256	264	272
6'3"	152	160	168	176	184	192	200	208	216	224	232	240	248	256	264	272	279
	Healthy Weight						Overweight						Obese				

Source: US Department of Health and Human Services, National Institutes of Health, National Health, Lung, and Blood Institute. The Clinical Guidelines on the Identification, Evaluation and Treatment of Overweight and Obesity in Adults: Evidence Report. September 1998 [NIH pub. No. 98-4083].

This table shows us that a woman who is 5 ft. 4 in. tall is considered overweight (BMI is 25 to 29) if she weighs between 145 and 169 pounds. She is considered obese (BMI is 30 or more) if she weighs 174 pounds or more. A man who is 5 ft. 10 in. tall is considered overweight (BMI is 25 to 29) if he weighs between 174 and 202 pounds, and is obese (BMI is 30 or more) if he weighs 209 pounds or more. You can also calculate your own BMI. The actual formula to determine BMI uses metric system measurements: weight in kilograms (kg) divided by height in meters, squared (m2).

When using pounds and inches, the formula needs to be altered slightly. Multiply your weight in pounds by 703. Divide that by your height in inches, squared:

BMI = (your weight in pounds x 703) ÷ (your height in inches x your height in inches)

For example, if you weigh 120 pounds and are 5 ft. 3 in. (63 in.) tall:

BMI = (120 x 703) ÷ (63 x 63) or 84,360 ÷ 3969 = 21.3

This is well within the healthy weight range.

Waist Size

Another important number to know is your waist size in inches. Having too much fat around your waist may increase health risks even more than having fat in other parts of your body. Women with a waist size of more than 35 inches and men with a waist size of more than 40 inches may have higher chances of developing diseases related to obesity.

Below are some numbers to aim for.

Measure	Target
Target BMI	18.5-24.9
Waist Size	Men: less than 40 in. Women: less than 35 in.
Blood Pressure	120/80 mm Hg or less
LDL (bad cholesterol)	Less than 100 mg/dl
HDL (good cholesterol)	Men: more than 40 mg/dl Women: more than 50 mg/dl
Triglycerides	Less than 150 mg/dl
Blood sugar (fasting)	Less than 100 mg/dl

For Women

Height (cm)	Height (inch)	Weight (Minimum) kg	Weight (Medium) kg	Weight (Maximum) kg
148	4'10''	44-48	46-51	49-57
150	4'11''	47-53	51-58	51-58
153	5'0''	46-50	49-54	52-59
155	5'1''	48-51	51-55	53-61
158	5'2''	49-53	52-57	55-63
160	5'3''	50-54	53-59	57-65
163	5'4''	52-56	54-61	59-66
165	5'5''	54-58	56-63	60-68
168	5'6''	55-69	58-65	62-70
170	5'7''	57-61	60-67	64-72
173	5'8''	59-63	62-69	66-74
175	5'9''	61-65	63-70	68-76
178	5'10''	63-67	65-72	69-79

For Men

Height (cm)	Height (inch)	Weight (Minimum) kg	Weight (Medium) kg	Weight (Maximum) kg
155	5'1''	51-54	54-59	57-64
158	5'2''	52-56	55-60	59-65
160	5'3''	53-57	56-62	60-67
163	5'4''	54-58	58-63	61-69
165	5'5''	56-60	59-65	63-71
168	5'6''	58-62	61-67	64-73
170	5'7''	60-64	63-69	67-75
173	5'8''	62-66	64-71	68-77
175	5'9''	64-68	66-73	70-79
178	5'10''	65-70	68-75	72-81
180	5'11''	67-72	70-77	74-84
183	6'0''	69-74	72-79	76-80
185	6'1''	71-76	71-76	78-88

2

INTRODUCTION TO YOGA

Yoga is a way of a better living. It ensures great or efficiency in work, and a better control over mind and emotions. Through yoga one can achieve both physical and mental harmony.

Yoga began as an ancient practice that originated in india circa 3000 B.C. Stone carved figures of yoga postures can be found in the Indus Valley depicting the original poses and practices. Yoga was part of the greater Hindu and Vedic tradition. Yoga can be traced back to the Ṛgveda itself, the oldest Hindu text which speaks about yoking our mind and insight to the Light of Truth or Reality. The history of Yoga is divided into five categories:

- ➤ Vedic period
- ➤ Pre-classical period
- ➤ Classical period
- ➤ Yoga in Medieval Times
- ➤ Yoga in Modern Times

One of the great Rṣis (Seers), Patańjali, compiled the essential features and principles of Yoga (which were earlier interspersed in Yoga Upaniṣads) in the form of 'Sūtras' (aphorisms) and made a vital contribution in the field of Yoga, nearly 4000 years ago (as dated by some famous western historians). According to Patańjali, Yoga is a conscious process of gaining mastery over the mind. The word **yoga** literally means "to yoke" or "union". More than just a practice of physical exercises, Yoga is the coming together of the individual self or consciousness, with the infinite universal consciousness or spirit. Yoga is a method of inquiry in to the nature of the mind, which emphasizes Pātańjala Yoga is one among the six systems of Indian philosophy known as Ṣaḍ darśanas.

The ultimate *"goal"* of yoga is to align to the universal consciousness in order to experience joy, freedom and the stillness of full consciousness. ***Alignment,*** is related to mind and body, and refers to how various parts of us are integrated and interconnected. The world is what think and believe it to be. It is subjective in essence - a projection of what we feel it is, based on past experiences and conditionings. What we see in others is what we have inside, like a mirror that is only projecting what is inside. We have the potential, using conscious intentions, thoughts and words, to co-create the life we want, to go beyond our limitations and fears, to surrender and open, to choose the type of person we want to be, to flow with the divine grace, to see the beauty in and all around us.

There are various paths of yoga that lead towards the ultimate goal of union, each a specialized branch of a comprehensive system, the main four being Karma Yoga, Bhakti Yoga, Raja Yoga and Jnana Yoga. Each, with their own world of techniques, supports people with different temperaments and approaches to life. All of the paths lead ultimately to the same destination - to union with Brahman/ God/ Oneness/ the Universe...- and the lessons from each need to be integrated if true wisdom is to be attained. The human personality can be divided broadly into four fundamental categories: emotional, active, intuitive and volitional. Patañjali has clearly understood this fact that each person has a different temperament and inclinations according to predominance of one or more of these categories. He, therefore, knew that the Yogic path had to be designed to suit the specific characteristics of an individual. Therefore, he suggests:

Raja Yoga – Path of Self - Discipline

Rajayoga is more popularly known as Ashtanga Yoga or the "eightfold path" that leads to spiritual liberation   Patañjali taught an eightfold (aṣṭāṇga) system of Yoga emphasizing an integral spiritual development. Ashtanga Yoga (Ashta

– 8, Anga – Limb) is the path to enlightenment that offers guidelines for a peaceful, meaningful and purposeful life.

The eight limbs of the Ashtanga Yoga are following ::

1. Yama.
2. Niyama.
3. Asana.
4. Pranayama.
5. Pratyahara.
6. Dharana.
7. Dyana.
8. Samadhi.

This constitutes a complete and integral system of spiritual training.

Bhakti Yoga – Path of Self-Surrender

Bhakti signifies both devotion and loving attachment to the Divine. Strictly the word denotes ' participation' (from the verbal root *bhaj* "to participate, to partake"). The Yogī on the devotional path literally participates in the Divine through surrender, devotion, service, worship and finally is drawn into mystical union with the Divine.

Jnana yoga – Path of Self-Awareness

Jñāna Yoga is the path of intellect and the path of analysis. This is also the Yoga of wisdom and has its own methodology. The methodology centers around hearing called as *śravaṇa*, recalling & analyzing called as *manana*, dwelling & meditating is *nididhyāsana*.

Karma Yoga – The Path of Selfless Action

The 4 major laws of *Karma Yoga* are described in Bhagavadgītā so that you can enjoy every moment of your work totally free from all stresses.

- ➢ work with a sense of duty;
- ➢ work without getting intensely attached (focussed attention) to the work;
- ➢ never allow the anxieties about the results interfere with your mind during the currency of the job;
- ➢ accept failure and success with equanimity.

Using these techniques of *Karma Yoga* we learn the art of 'working in relaxation' with total 'Awareness in Action' . Not losing sight of the innate bliss and poise, the path of work teaches us to interact in society judiciously and effectively.

So, as you practice Yoga, it does not only help you to improve your physical body but also helps in maintaining your inner peace and realaxing your mind. Thus there is nothing that yoga will not help. Moreover yoga is not just a one day practice; it is a life loong commitment.

3

BASIC GUIDELINES

Before begin your yoga practice you have to follow this guidelines .There are many principles in yogaasana from many traditions. Here are just a few very basic ideas to keep in mind throughout your practice:

If you have a medical condition you should consult your medical or health specialist before embarking on this Slimming Yoga program. It also applies to pregnant women and children below 12 years old.

Time to practice

Put aside a specific time in your day to enjoy your Yoga practice. Dawn and dusk are considered the best times of the day to practice Yoga, as the rising and setting of the sun charge our body with special energy. However, if these times are impossible for you, find another time of the day that works best for you and practice consistently. Practice in the morning if you want to prepare your mind and body for the day, and charge your body with positive energy. Keep in mind that in the morning or in cold weather your muscles will be stiffer, so ease carefully into the postures at first. Practice in the evening if you want to relax after a stressful day, unwind and centre. In the evenings your body will be more flexible, so you'll be able to go deeper into postures.

Place for practice

Find a place where you are least likely to be disturbed. It can be your room, garden or beach - indoors or outdoors, wherever there is an even, flat surface. If you are practicing indoors, make sure that the room is ventilated and with comfortable temperature. Air conditioned rooms are not advisable - when the environment is cold your body is stiff, and muscles stretch slowly. A clean environment and fresh air adds additional benefits to the breathing practice. Make sure that you have enough space to allow you to move around, and extend the arms and legs freely. Turn your phone off and hang a note on your door to say that you are having time to yourself.

Eating and Drinking

Never practice directly after eating. Yoga should be done on empty stomach. Therefore allow at least 1 hour after a snack and 2 - 3 hours after a heavy meal before you begin your practice. It is best to drink before or after your Yoga session, to avoid becoming dehydrated. Try to avoid drinking water during the practice, to avoid losing your concentration on Yoga postures and breathing. However if you are practicing in the morning, have at least a glass of warm water before your practice, or a light snack (fruit or yoghurt). When you finish your practice eat a proper breakfast.

What to Wear

Wear comfortable, light, loose clothing, preferably made of natural fibers. Your clothes should not restrict your movements. Remove your jewelry, watch and spectacles if possible. Yoga is practiced with bare feet.

What You Need

Get a special Yoga mat for yourself. It provides padding as well as a non-slip surface to practice on, and makes your practice easier and safer. You can find one in any sports shop. No one else should use your mat. This is not only for hygiene reasons, but also because you will eventually build up energy on your mat that will support you throughout the Yoga practice. You can also get a cushion to make your meditation more comfortable and a blanket if you wish to cover yourself while relaxing in the Corpse Pose at the end of the session. If you want, you can play relaxing, soothing music in the background - just make sure it's not too loud.

How To Practice

Perform all the postures slowly and with control. You are not in competition with anyone, not even yourself. You'll progress faster when you take things slowly.

❖ Concentrate on your breathing, feel the air slowly flowing through your body, relaxing and energizing it.
❖ Relax. Let go of any unnecessary tension, stress or negative thoughts.
❖ Start every session with the warm-up. It's essential to avoid injuries.
❖ Modify the postures for your body. The instructions and pictures of the yoga postures in this book are the final goal - the direction you are going towards, not where you need to be after your first few sessions. Experiment and explore different positions and alignments to make the posture work for your body.
❖ Don't expect instant results. Yoga is a not a quick fix for your weight problems. Patience is a key to unlocking the long-term slimming benefits of Yoga.
❖ Have Fun! The best way to get results with your Yoga practice is to enjoy it. Feeling happy while practicing Yoga puts the mind and body into a positive state.
❖ Most Importantly, listen to and respect your body. Never force any movement. Let your body lead you, it is your greatest teacher!

Alignment of the Physical Body:

❖ **Spine**

Yoga asana focuses on elongating the spine and increasing its range of motion. Because Yoga is ultimately of practice of working with subtle energies, maintaining alignment and length in the Spine is of the utmost importance in yoga asana alignment.

❖ Hands /Feet: Our foundation

We begin by setting up and aligning the foundation of the poses. Spread your hands / feet wide to create the most stable foundation possible to support our being, plant down through the 4 corners of your hands and feet, especially the big toes, then draw the energy in and up through the body though the domes or "nostrils" of the hands and feet. *Mantra: Spread out. Plant Down. Draw in.*

❖ Soft Elbows / Knees

There are no straight lines in nature and thus considering we are a creation of nature, this goes for our bodies as well. We can always maintain softness in these joints, ensuring that we are not hyper-extending, as this compromises the integrity of alignment in the pose. Teachers will often remind us to "micro-bend" or to have soft elbows and knees as this helps us to yield into the earth or whatever surface we are upon. Actively yielding to the Earth creates a rebound effect, elongating the body upwards into space.

❖ Shoulders / Hips

These are the gateways for the arms and legs to connect with the torso, and two common areas in which we commonly experience tension in the body. When the shoulders are hugging the ears, the body is being sent messages of stress! So think about relaxing and softening the shoulder, rolling your shoulders away from your ears creating as much space as possible in the neck. Keep the hips level, ensuring that their height is equalized.

❖ Neutralize Pelvic tilt

Think of the pelvis as a bowl filled with water. In standing and balancing positions, we want to keep the bowl level so that we arenot tipping forward and hyper arching our low back, spilling the water out the front, or tilting it too far up, as is common in people with tight hips doing seated postures, spilling the water out the back. Make sure the hips and pelvis are level. If you find your low back rounding and your pelvis tipping up, then help yourself to a cushion or two or three so that you can be aligned and comfortable. We also want to make sure we neutralize the front to back placement of the hips so that it rests just atop the legs.

❖ **Neck and head**

In most active styles of yoga asana, the general principle is to keep the head and neck long and in line with the spine, bringing the chin back in if are heads are jutting forward. I know a body worker who tells his clients: "Take the head away from the computer! .

❖ **Soft Face & Eyes**

Make sure your eyes are soft, your jaw is relaxed and soft, and your face is nice and released. Having a soft controlled gaze or focus, or Drishti, helps us to develop concentration, and focused consciousness to see the world as it is. When we are beginning our practice of yoga, we often lose balance by looking around and paying attention to all of the stimulation and distraction outside of ourselves. Focusing the attention inwards, by holding a soft gaze point either to our 3rd eye or our hearts, encourage stability and inward looking.

Tips for Transitioning between Poses in Alignment:

- Connect and synchronize movements with the breath
- Breathe into the back body while transitioning
- Move with steady graceful flowing rhythm
- Maintain steady moment to moment awareness
- Take your time and move from stability and integration first
- Activate stability before active expansion
- Adjust alignment of back leg first, then front leg

Asana and the Breath

Inhale When...

- ❖ Opening, unfolding, expanding outer body
- ❖ Lengthening and opening the spine
- ❖ Opening the arms to the sides or overhear
- ❖ Coming out of forward folds of lateral standing poses
- ❖ Going up into a pose against gravity -bringing lightness to a pose

Exhale When...

- ❖ Closing, unfolding, or flexing the outer body
- ❖ Bringing the arms to the midline
- ❖ Going into forward folds of lateral bends
- ❖ Releasing down with gravity
- ❖ Twisting

4

SURYANAMASKARA

Suryanamaskar is an ancient method yogic method to worship Sun. In Sanskrit literature surya means sun, and the word namaskara means salutation. Therefore, this practice is known as the ¬Suryanamaskar|| or 'salutation to the sun'. Suryanamaskara was developed in Indian subcontinent thousands of years ago by a great sage Patanjali and their desciples,They advised all human beings to practice these yogic methods in front of the sun in their daily life for good health, illumination, mental and physical stabilitiy.

Surya Namaskar is one of the best exercises that people can perform. The benefits accruing from these exercises are unique and excellent. This is a yoga based exercise and it is customary to perform Surya Namaskar after performing loosening yoga exercises. The Surya Namaskar is performed usually early in the morning facing the morning rising Sun.
Surya Namaskara is a set of 12 Asanas (postures), , each posture having its own breathing pattern (inhalation or exhalation), and its own mantra.
Its revitalizes each and every cell of the body, gives physical strength, flexibility, and mental calmness.

Benefits of Surya Namaskara

- ❖ It helps to keep you disease=-free and healthy.
- ❖ Helps to lose weight.
- ❖ Helps to get a glowing skin
- ❖ Regular practice promotes balance in the body.
- ❖ Improves blood circulation.
- ❖ Strengthens the heart.

- ❖ Tones the digestive tract.
- ❖ Stimulate abdominal muscles respiratory systemm, lymphatic system. Spinal nerves and other internal organs.
- ❖ Tones the spine,neck,shoulder arm,hands wrist,back and leg muscles thereby promoting overall flexibility.
- ❖ Psychologically, it regulates the interconnectedness of body,breath and mind thus making you calmer and boosting the energy level with sharpened awareness.
- ❖

SURYA NAMASKARA

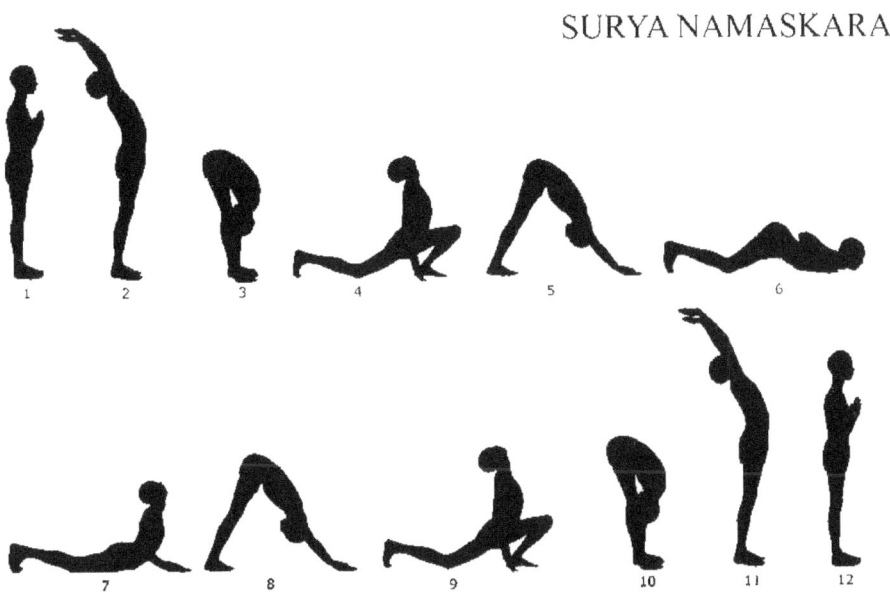

Pranamasana (Prayer pose) – 1st & 12th Pose

Pranamasana or the Prayer Pose is the starting and twelfth pose for Surya Namaskara. In Sanskrit the word _Pranam ' means _to pay respect '; so this asana known as Pranamasana. Method: Stand erect with folded hands close to the chest and palms are held together in the form of prayer pose. Look straight ahead, Exhale the breath normally. Benefits: It creates a sense of relaxation, calmness and concentration in the mind at beginning the Surya Namaskara.

Hasta Uttanasana (Raised arms pose)- 2nd & 11th pose

Hasta Uttanasana or the raised arms pose is part of the Surya Namaskara series of asanas come at 2nd and the 11th steps. Method: Raise both the hands up above the crown from Pranamasana pose. Inhale the breath normally while raising your hands. Bend the trunk and neck slightly backward. Benefits: It improves digestive process; It strengthens and tones the abdominal and chest musculature. It supports respiratory system too.

Padahastasana (Hand to Foot pose)- 3rd & 10th pose

Padahastasana or the Hand to Foot pose is part of the Surya Namaskara series of asanas come at 3rd and the 10th steps. Method: Bend forward from Hasta Uttanasana pose and try to touch the floor with your both hands. Exhales breathe normally while bending forward. Benefits: Padahastasana makes the body flexible and strengthen, helps to decrease excess abdominal fat and very beneficial for the gastrointestinal and nervous system.

Ashwa Sanchalanasana (The Equestrian Pose) – 4th & 9th pose

Ashwa Sanchalanasana or the Equestrian pose is part of the Surya Namaskara series of asanas come at 4th and the 9th steps. Method: Stretch the left leg as far back as possible from Padahastasana pose while inhaling the breath normally. At the same time, bend the right knee. While looking straight ahead the hands should be kept straight with fingers touching the floor. Arch the back a little with head tilted back. The same steps should be repeated with left knee in the second round of Surya Namaskara. Benefits: Ashwa Sanchalanasana tones the abdominal organs, It gives flexibility to the body and balances central nervous system.

Parvatasana (The Mountain Pose) – 5th & 8th pose

Parvatasana or the Mountain pose is part of the Surya Namaskara series of asanas and come at 5th and the 8th step. In Sanskrit terminology, ‐Parvata ' means mountain and this pose looks like a mountain so it is known as Parvatasana. Method: While exhaling, take the right leg backward from Ashwa Sanchalanasana pose and place it parallel to the left leg, raise the buttocks at the same time. Place the hands straight supporting the weight of the body. The head should be placed between the hands. Benefits: Parvatasana strengthens the muscles of both upper and lower limbs, maintains the blood circulation to Central nervous system and tones peripheral nervous system.

Ashtanga Namaskara (Eight-Limbed salutation) – 6th pose

Ashtanga Namaskara or the Eight-Limbed salutation is part of the Surya Namaskara series of asanas come at 6th step. In this pose, the body touches the ground in eight locations –the head, the chest, the two palms, the two knees, and the two toes. In Sanskrit grammar, ‐ashta|| means eight and ‐anga|| means part. Hence this asana is known as Ashtanga Namaskara. Method: Lower the body to the ground from Parvatasana pose in such a way that it touches the floor at eight locations – the head, the chest, the two palms, the two knees, and the two toes, Suspended the breath for a while. Try to lift other parts in air. Benefits: It strengthens the muscles of the both upper and lower limbs and strengthens respiratory system.

Bhujangasana (The Cobra Pose)- 7th pose

Bhujangasana is also famous as a cobra pose in yoga. The meaning of _ Bhujanga ' in Sanskrit means _cobra ' snake and _Asana ' means _Pose '. In this asana person 's head and trunk resembles a cobra with raised hood, hence the name Bhujangasana. It is a major backward bending asanas used in yoga. It appears as the 7th pose in the Surya Namaskara series asanas. Method: While inhaling raise the body by using the hands from Ashtanga Namaskara pose. Arch your head backward. This position looks like the cobra which has raised its hood. Benefits: Bhujangasana strengthens the whole back musculature especially lower back, It improves the flexibility of the spine and surrounding muscles, good for the gastrointestinal, reproductive and urogenital system.

5

YOGASANA

Asana is roughly translated from Sanskrit as "pose" or "posture." This simply means a *"yoga pose."* The literal translation actually means *"to be in a comfortable seated position."* This comes from the branch of yoga called ashtanga yoga, and it refers to the physical exertion and also the mental relaxation that happens in yoga. Practicing these asanas will bring you awareness both internally and externally.Many of the poses below have the instructions to "repeat on the other side." This means that it is a two-sided pose, and it only works muscles in one side of the body at a time. Always repeat the pose on both sides of the body to build strength and flexibility equally in the body.

Prasarita Padottanasana

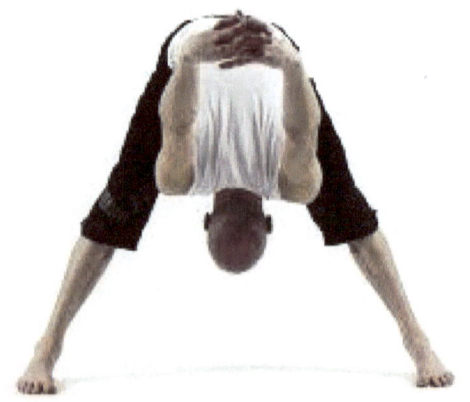

The series of Prasarita Padottanasana designed to stretch and strengthen the body. Known for its revitalizing effect, this forward Bend is also a version of semi-inverted pose and helps to make the life of the practitioner simpler and smoother. The Wide-Legged Forward Bend gets its name from Sanskrit to English translation, where 'Prasarita' means Wide or Stretched Out, 'Pada' means foot, 'Ut' means intense, 'Tan' means stretch and 'Asana' means Pose. A centerfold in the league of Ashtanga Yoga Primary series, Wide-Legged Forward Bend Pose is a part of the standing forward pose and targets a practitioner's entire body. Those practitioners who practice intense backbends can use Prasarita Padottanasana to counterbalance the backbends and bring a sense of harmony. We have put together a list of benefits offered by Prasarita Padottanasana which will help you to understand why it is important and must be added to any sequence on a regular basis.

❖ Stretching the Lower body
❖ Refreshing the mind
❖ Lower Backache reliever
❖ Helping the digestion.
❖ Creating better posture
❖ Activating the Energy Center

Traditionally, your hands should be touching the floor in front of you in this pose, but we like the extra shoulder stretch! Spread your feet 3-4 feet apart, and bend forward at the HIPS, not the waist. This means that your back should be as straight as possible when you bend, and you should not simply "hunch" forward. If you're bending properly, you will actually feel a strong stretch in the hamstrings. Practice in front of the mirror to try to get the correct form.

Hold for 5-6 breaths. If you feel comfortable enough, clasp the hands behind the back. Try to bring them up towards the ceiling to give the arms and shoulders an extra stretch.

Sarvangasana

Sarvangasana or shoulder stand is a yoga pose wherein the whole body is balanced on the shoulders. It is also a part of the Padma Sadhana yoga sequence. 'Sarv' means all, 'anga' means part of a body, and 'asana' is posture. As the name indicates, Sarvangasana influences the functioning of all parts of your body. This asana is highly beneficial in maintaining the mental and physical health and is also referred as 'Queen of asanas' .

Benefits of Sarvangasana :

- ❖ Stimulates the thyroid and parathyroid glands and normalizes their functions
- ❖ Strengthens the arms and shoulders and keeps the spine flexible
- ❖ Nourishes the brain with more blood
- ❖ Stretches the heart muscles by returning more venous blood to the heart
- ❖ Brings relief from constipation, indigestion and varicose veins

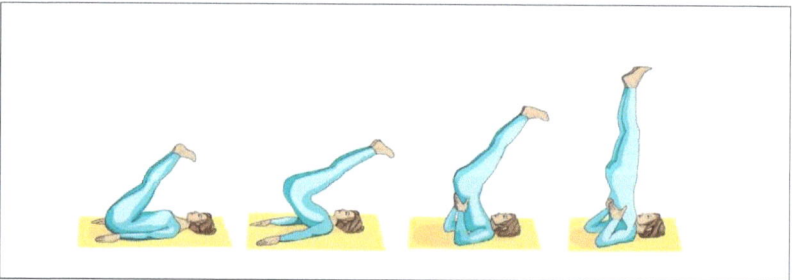

This is considered an inversion because your body is upside down! Inversions such as headstand, forearm stand, and handstand can make yoga practice very fun! Begin with your back on the ground, your knees slightly bent, and your feet in the air. Press your hands flat on the ground, and use them to roll yourself backward on your upper back. As you do this, bring the hands to your lower back, just above your hips, to keep yourself upright. Slowly extend your legs toward the ceiling.

Beginner Modification: If you're having difficulty staying up, place your hands on your hips to help support your weight better.Hold for 5-6 breaths, and work towards 30 seconds.

Paschimottanasana

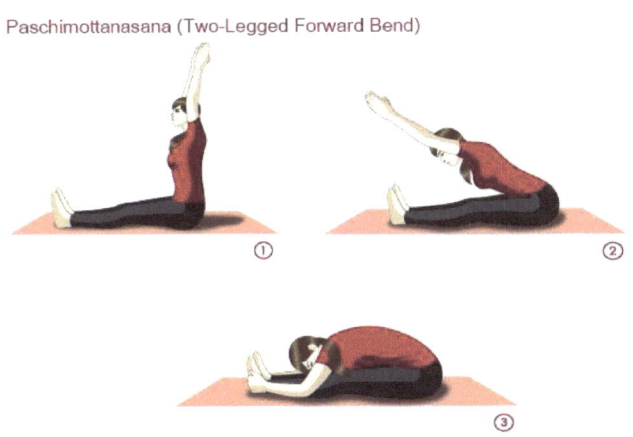

Paschimottanasana (Two-Legged Forward Bend)

This asana gives the back part of the body a good stretch, all the way from the ankles to the head. The muscles of the anterior part of the body are contracted, and this creates pressure on the abdomen and thorax, thereby, improving respiratory functions and the functioning of the intra-abdominal glands, specifically focusing on secretions. The flexibility in the lumbar region, the thighs, and the hips is improved. There is an enhancement in the circulation of the blood in the back, and the nerves of the spinal cord are toned. This asana also helps reduce fat in the hips, thighs, and abdomen region. This asana purifies the Nadis and also stimulates the Kundalini Shakti.

Sit erect, with your legs, stretched out in front of you. Make sure that your toes are flexed towards you. Inhale and raise your arms over your head. Stretch. Exhale and bend forward. Feel the fold from your hip joints. Your chin should move towards your toes. Stretch out your arms, and let them reach the furthest they can, possibly till your toes. But make sure that you don't stretch too far. Inhale. Then, lifting your head slightly, elongate your spine. Exhale and move your navel towards your knees. Repeat this a few times. Then, place your head on your legs, and hold the pose. Inhale and come up back to the sitting position with your arms stretched out. Exhale and lower your arms.

Halasana

Practicing this asana regularly rejuvenates and nurtures your entire body. Halasana increases the blood flow and the suppleness in the lumbar and thoracic regions in the body, and also releases stress and tension in the throat and neck. If there is an accumulation of mucous or phlegm in the respiratory system or the sinuses, this asana helps to flush it all out. With regular practice, your breath will also be streamlined.

Halasana heals and calms the sympathetic nervous system. It helps to balance the secretions in the glands, specifically thyroxine and adrenaline. It also removes toxins from the urinary and digestive tracts. If you have had a history of high blood pressure, this asana helps relieve hypertension as well.

Lie flat on your back, with your arms placed beside your body and your palms facing downwards.Inhale, and lift your feet off the ground using your abdominal muscles. Your legs should be at a 90-degree angle. Use your hands to support your hips and lift them off the floor. Bring your feet in an 180-degree angle, such that your toes are placed over and beyond your head. Make sure your back is perpendicular to the ground. Hold the position for a minute while focusing on your breathing. Exhale, and gently bring down your legs. Avoid jerking your legs while releasing the pose

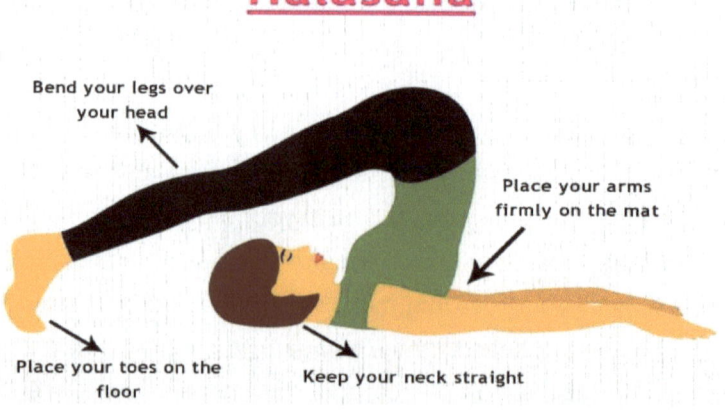

Halasana

Bend your legs over your head

Place your arms firmly on the mat

Place your toes on the floor

Keep your neck straight

Shirsasna

Shirsasna Increases blood supply to the head, therefore is beneficial for brain function and all sensory organs in the head (eyes, ears etc.). Improves memory and the ability to concentrate. This Asana stimulates and regulates all the body's systems. Helps to counter problems related to menopause.

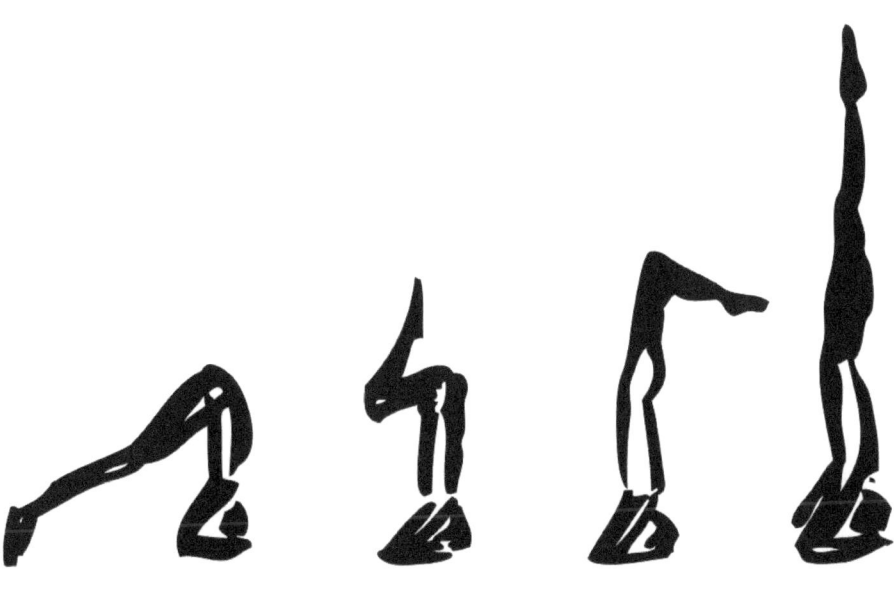

Sit in Vajrasana. Hands rest on the thighs. >Breathing normally place the head on the floor in front of the knees. Clasp the fingers behind the head and support the back of the head with the clasped hands. The forearms rest on the floor and the elbows form an equilateral triangle with the head. >Tuck the toes under, lift the hips and straighten the legs. Concentrate on the balance of the body. Walk the feet in closer to the body so that the buttocks are high above the head. Transfer the weight of the body onto the forearms and raise the feet from the floor. Keeping the back straight bring the heels towards the buttocks. Finally, straighten the legs fully upright and allow the feet to remain relaxed.

Balance the body weight between forearms, head and neck in a relaxed manner. >Hold the posture as long as possible, but not more than five minutes. >Slowly lower the legs by bending the knees and bringing the feet towards the buttocks and then the toes to the floor. >Relax forward for some time in Yoga Mudra and then return to Vajrasana.

Sethu Bandhasana

This asana gets its name from the Sanskrit words   'Setu' , which means bridge, 'Bandha' , which means lock, and   'Asana' , which means pose. This pose resembles the structure of a bridge, and therefore, it is named as such. This pose stretches your back, neck, and chest and relaxes your body.

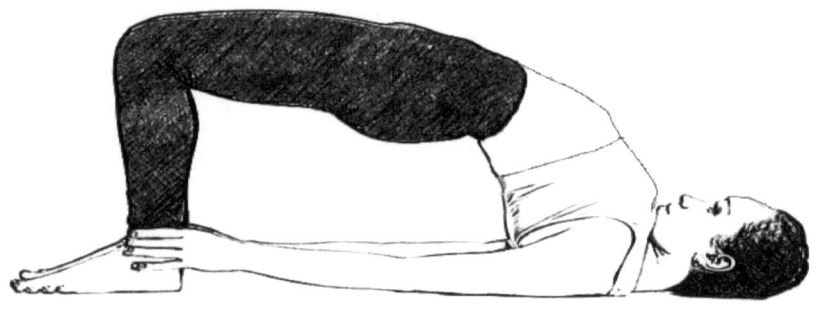

To begin, lie on your back.Fold your knees and keep your feet hip distance apart on the floor, 10-12 inches from your pelvis, with knees and ankles in a straight line. Keep your arms beside your body, palms facing down. Inhaling, slowly lift your lower back, middle back and upper back off the floor; gently roll in the shoulders; touch the chest to the chin without bringing the chin down, supporting your weight with your shoulders, arms and feet. Feel your bottom firm up in this pose. Both the thighs are parallel to each other and to the floor. If you wish, you could interlace the fingers and push the hands on the floor to lift the torso a little more up, or you could support your back with your palms. Keep breathing easily. Hold the posture for a minute or two and exhale as you gently release the pose.

Benefits of Sethu Bandhasana :

- Strengthens the back muscles.
- Relieves the tired back instantaneously.
- Gives a good stretch to the chest, neck and spine.
- Calms the brain, reducing anxiety, stress and depression.
- Opens up the lungs and reduces thyroid problems.
- Helps improve digestion.
- Helps relieve the symptoms of menopause and menstrual pain.
- Helpful in asthma, high blood pressure, osteoporosis, and sinusitis.

Vasisthasana

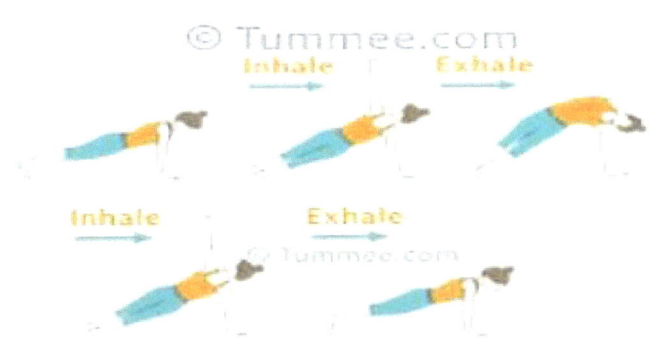

Perform Adho Mukha Svanasana. Shift onto the outside edge of your left foot, and stack your right foot on top of the left. Now swing your right hand onto your right hip, turn your torso to the right as you do, and support the weight of your body on the outer left foot and left hand.Make sure that the supporting hand isn't directly below its shoulder; position the hand slightly in front of its shoulder, so the supporting arm is angled a bit relative to the floor. Straighten the arm by firming the triceps muscle, and press the base of the index finger firmly against the floor.Firm the scapulas and sacrum against the back torso. Strengthen the thighs, and press through the heels toward the floor. Align your entire body into one long diagonal line from the heels to the crown.If you'd like you can stretch the top arm toward the ceiling, parallel to the line of the shoulders. Keep the head in a neutral position, or turn it to gaze up at the top hand.Stay in this position for 15 to 30 seconds. Come back to Adho Mukha Svanasana, take a few breaths, and repeat to the right side for the same length of time. Then return to Adho Mukha Svanasana for a few more breaths, and finally release into Balasana.

Benefits :

- ❖ Strengthens the arms, belly, and legs
- ❖ Stretches and strengthens the wrists
- ❖ Stretches the backs of the legs (in the full version described below)
- ❖ Improves sense of balance

Pavanamukthasana

The Wind-Relieving Pose is a reclined posture that is suitable for everyone, whether they are beginners or advanced practitioners. This pose helps to release digestive gases from the intestines and stomach with great ease. It is also called the One-Legged Knee-to-Chest Pose. It is best to practice this asana first thing every morning so that all the trapped gases in your digestive tract are released. This should also be one of the first asanas you practice as once the gases are released, it will make practicing other asanas easier. Yoga must be practiced at least four to six hours after a meal, when your stomach and bowels are both empty.

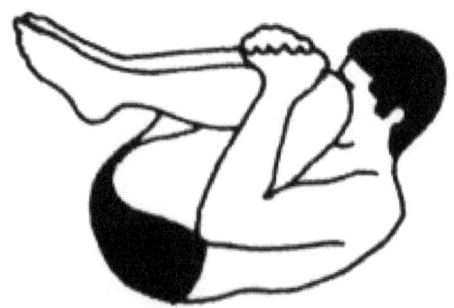

Lie flat on your back on a smooth surface, ensuring that your feet are together, and your arms are placed beside your body. Take a deep breath. As you exhale, bring your knees towards your chest, and press your thighs on your abdomen. Clasp your hands around your legs as if you are hugging your knees. Hold the asana while you breathe normally. Every time you exhale, make sure you tighten the grip of the hands on the knee, and increase the pressure on your chest. Every time you inhale, ensure that you loosen the grip. Exhale and release the pose after you rock and roll from side to side about three to five times. Relax.

Benefits :

- It strengthens the abdominal muscles and massages the intestines and internal organs of the digestive system, therefore releasing trapped gases and improving digestion.
- It strengthens the back muscles and tones the muscles of the arms and the legs.
- It improves the circulation of blood in the hip area.
- It eases the tension in the lower back.
- It stimulates the reproductive organs and massages the pelvic muscles. It also helps to cure menstrual disorders.
- It helps burn fat in the thighs, buttocks, and abdominal area.
- It helps to stretch the back and neck.

Veerabadhrasana

This pose strengthens the arms, shoulders, thighs and back muscles, all in one go. This pose is named after *Veerabhadra,* a fierce warrior, an incarnation of Lord Shiva. The story of the **warrior Veerabhadra**, as all stories from Upanishads, has a moral that adds value to our life.

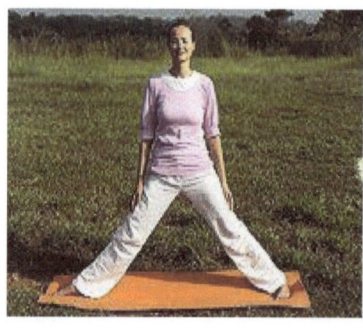 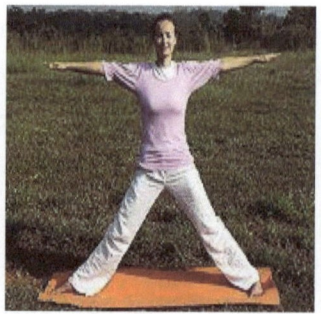 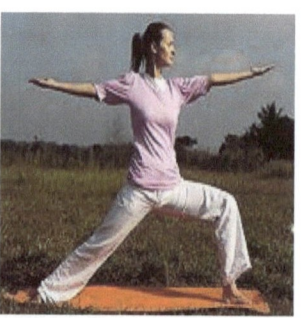

Veera - vigorous, warrior, courageous; *Bhadra* - good, auspicious; *Asana* - Posture.Stand straight with your legs wide apart by a distance of at least 3-4 feet. Turn your right foot out by 90 degrees and left foot in by about 15 degrees. Checkpoint: Is the heel of the right foot aligned to the center of the left foot?.Lift both arms sideways to shoulder height with your palms facing upwards. Checkpoint: Are your arms parallel to the ground?. Breathing out, bend your right knee. Checkpoint: Are your right knee and right ankle forming a straight line? Ensure that your knee does not overshoot the ankle. Turn your head and look to your right. As you settle down in the yoga posture stretch your arms further. Make a gentle effort to push your pelvis down. Hold the yoga posture with the determination of a warrior. Smile like a happy smiling warrior. Keep breathing as you go down. Breathing in, come up. Breathing out, bring your hands down from the sides. Repeat the yoga posture for the left side (turn your left foot out by 90 degrees and turn the right foot in by about 15 degrees).

Benefits :

- ❖ Strengthens and tones the arms, legs and lower back.
- ❖ Improves balance in the body, helps increase stamina.
- ❖ Beneficial for those with sedentary or deskbound jobs.
- ❖ Extremely beneficial in case of frozen shoulders.
- ❖ Releases stress in the shoulders very effectively in a short span of time.
- ❖ Brings auspiciousness, courage, grace and peace.

Bhujangasana

The Cobra pose or Bhujangasana is a basic Hatha yoga pose, and as such, is very often practiced either on its own, or as part of the Sun Salutations.

Bhujanga means snake in Sanskrit, and in this pose we imitate a snake lifting its head while working the shoulders, upper back and spine. The Bhujangasana is also believed to be a great aid for the digestive fire, helping to purify the body.

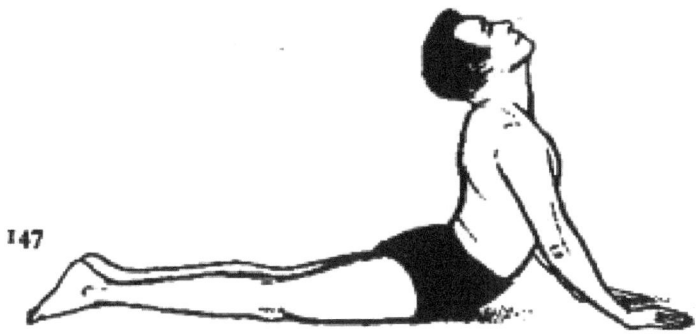

147

To start the pose, lie on your stomach and place your forehead on the floor. You can have your feet together, or hip width apart. Keep the tops of your feet pressing against the floor. Place your hands underneath your shoulders, keeping your elbows close to your body. Draw your shoulder blades back and down, and try to maintain this throughout the pose. Draw your pubic bone towards the floor to stabilize your lower back, and press your feet actively onto the floor. With the next inhale, start lifting your head and chest off the floor. Be mindful of opening the chest, and don't place all of your weight onto your hands. Keep the elbows lightly bent and keep the back muscles working. Take your hands off from the floor for a moment to see what is a comfortable, maintainable height for you. Keep your shoulders relaxed. With exhale lower yourself back onto the ground. Take 2-3 rounds of inhaling yourself up into the cobra, and exhaling down to the floor. Then hold for 2-3 full breaths, and come back down. Rest on the floor for a few breaths, or enjoy Child's pose as a gentle counter pose.

Dhanurasana

Dhanurasana or the Bow Pose is one of the 12 basic Hatha Yoga poses. It is also one of the three main back stretching exercises. It gives the entire back a good stretch, thus imparting flexibility as well as strength to the back.

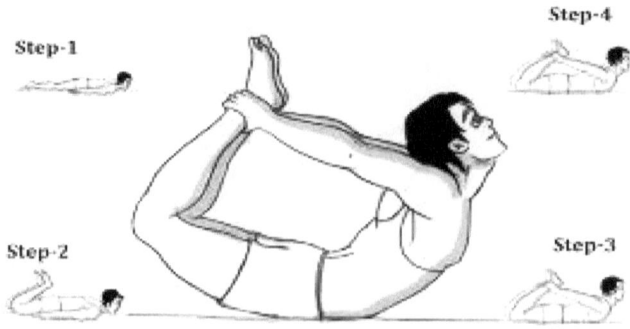

DHANURASANA (BOW POSE)

Lie on your stomach with your feet hip-width apart and your arms by the side of your body. Fold your knees, take your hands backwards and hold your ankles. Breathing in, lift your chest off the ground and pull your legs up and back. Look straight ahead with a smile on your face. Keep the pose stable while paying attention to your breath. Your body is now curved and taut as a bow. Continue to take long deep breaths as you relax in this pose. But bend only as far as your body permits you to. Do not overdo the stretch. After 15 -20 seconds, as you exhale, gently bring your legs and chest to the ground. Release the ankles and relax.

Benefits :

- Strengthens the back and abdominal muscles
- Stimulates the reproductive organs
- Opens up the chest, neck and shoulders
- Tones the leg and arm muscles
- Adds greater flexibility to the back
- Good stress and fatigue buster
- Relieves menstrual discomfort and constipation

- Helps people with renal (kidney) disorders

Shalabhasana

In Sanskrit the word "Shalabh" stands for Locust or grasshopper which is a one type of insect, basically found in grass. While doing Shalabhasana the complete body shape seems like a locust or grasshopper structure thus this posture is additionally known as Locust pose. Shalabhasana advantages to strengthen back muscles and curing ailments like sciatica and back ache. There are total three methods for practicing Shalabhasana. We describe these methods one by one in a correct manner. This Asana is simple to do and suitable for everybody. This is the special Asana for the spine.

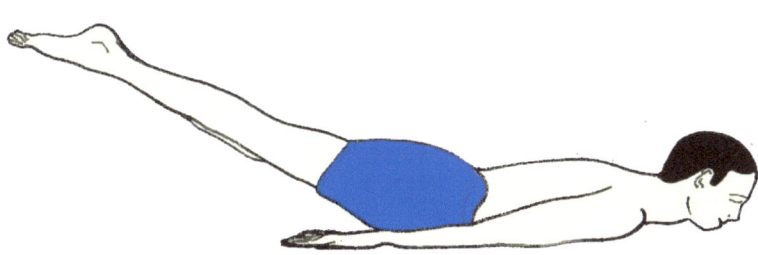

Method 1 :

Lie down on your Stomach; place both hands underneath the thighs. Breath in (inhale) and lift your right leg up, (your leg should not bend at the knee). Your chin should rest on the ground. Hold this position about ten to twenty seconds. After that exhale and take down your leg in the initial position. Similarly do it with your left leg. Repeat this for five to seven times. After doing it with the left leg, inhale and lift your both legs up (Your legs should not bend at the knees; lift your legs as much as you can). With both legs repeat the process for two to four times.

Method 2 :

Lie down on your stomach; straighten your right hand while touching the head and the ear. (Keep your right hand straight in the ground in resting position).

Keep your left hand on the back. Now inhale; lift your head and your right hand up along with lift your left leg above the ground level. Hold this position for some time. After exhale and slowly- slowly come back to normal position. Similarly repeat this process with your alternate hands and legs.

Method 3 :

Lie down on your stomach. Take your both hands behind and hold the wrists of one hand with the other. Now inhale; at first lift your chest as much as you can and look upwards. Slowly lift your body from the both sides. Now exhale and come back to your initial position.

Benefits :

- ❖ It is beneficial in all the disorders at the lower end of the spine.
- ❖ Most helpful for backache and sciatica pain.
- ❖ Useful for removing unwanted fats around abdomen, waist, hips and thighs.
- ❖ Daily practice of this Asana can cures cervical spondylitis and spinal cord ailments.
- ❖ Strengthening your wrists, hips, thighs, legs, buttocks, lower abdomen and diaphragm.
- ❖ Toughens back muscles.

Trikonasana

This asana resembles a triangle, and therefore, is named so. The name comes from the Sanskrit words trikona, meaning triangle, and asana, meaning posture. This asana is known to stretch the muscles and improve the regular bodily functions. Unlike most other yoga asanas, this requires you to keep your eyes open while you practice it to maintain balance.

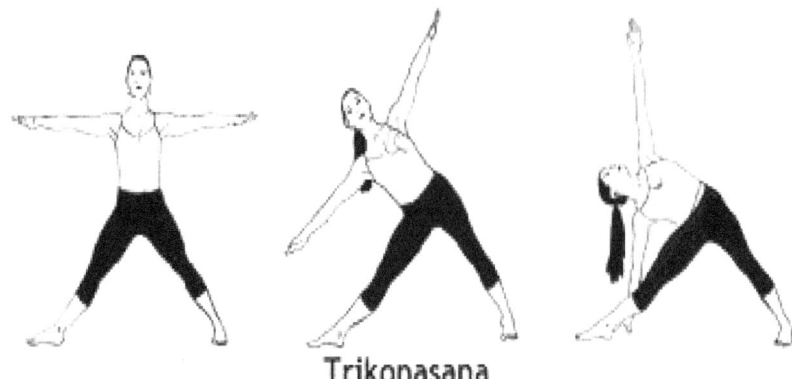

Trikonasana

Stand straight. Separate your feet comfortably wide apart (about 31/2 to 4 feet). Turn your right foot out 90 degrees and left foot in by 15 degrees. Now align the center of your right heel with the center of your arch of left foot. Ensure that your feet are pressing the ground and the weight of your body is equally balanced on both the feet. Inhale deeply and as you exhale, bend your body to the right, downward from the hips, keeping the waist straight, allowing your left hand to come up in the air while your right hand comes down towards floor. Keep both arms in straight line. Rest your right hand on your shin, ankle, or the floor outside your right foot, whatever is possible without distorting the sides of the waist. Stretch your left arm toward the ceiling, in line with the tops of your shoulders. Keep your head in a neutral position or turn it to the left, eyes gazing softly at the left palm. Ascertain that your body is bent sideways and not backward or forward. Pelvis and chest are wide open. Stretch maximum and be steady. Keep taking in long deep breaths. With each exhalation, relax the body more and more. Just be with the body and the breath. As you inhale, come up, bring your arms down to your sides, and straighten your feet. Repeat the same on the other side.

Benefits :

- Strengthens the legs, knees, ankles, arms and chest
- Stretches and opens the hips, groins, hamstrings, calves, shoulders, chest and spine
- Increases mental and physical equilibrium
- Helps improve digestion
- Reduces anxiety, stress, back pain and sciatica

Noukasana

Naukasana comes from the two Sanskrit words 'nauka' which means 'boat' and 'asana' meaning 'posture' or 'seat'. It is a posture in which our body takes the shape of a boat. If you have always had a problem losing the extra paunch in your stomach area, then this asana is good for those who wish to reduce belly fat as well as to tone the abs.

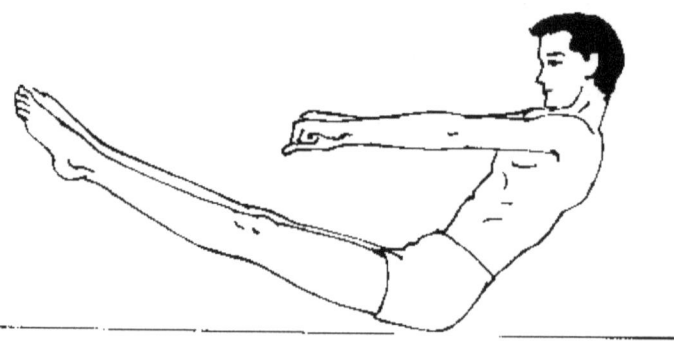

Lie on your back with your feet together and arms beside your body. Take a deep breath in and as you exhale, lift your chest and feet off the ground, stretching your arms towards your feet. Your eyes, fingers and toes should be in a line. Feel the tension in your navel area as the abdominal muscles contract. Keep breathing deeply and easily while maintaining the pose. As you exhale, come back to the ground slowly and relax.

Benefits :

- ❖ Strengthens the back and abdominal muscles
- ❖ Tones the leg and arm muscles
- ❖ Useful for people with hernia

6

PRANAYAMA

Yoga breathing exercises, also known as pranayama, are an important part of a developing yoga practice. Pranayama is one of the Eight Limbs of Yoga referenced by *The Yoga Sutras of Patanjali,* which means that it was considered an integral step on the path to enlightenment. In addition to supporting and deepening your yoga asana practice, learning ways to calm or invigorate the body through breathing will greatly benefit all aspects of your life. Paying attention to the breath is also a meditation technique that can be used on or off the mat, as it has the effect of keeping us constantly in the present moment. The past and the future melt away when the mind becomes fully focused on breathing.

Pranayama is loosely translated as prana or breath control. The ancient yogis developed many breathing techniques to maximize the benefits of prana. Pranayama is used in yoga as a separate practice to help clear and cleanse the body and mind. It is also used in preparation for meditation, and in asana,the practice of postures, to help maximize the benefits of the practice, and focus the mind. Breathing is so simple and so obvious we often take it for granted, ignoring the power it has to affect body, mind and spirit. With each inhale we bring oxygen into the body and spark the transformation of nutrients into fuel. Each exhale purges the body of carbon dioxide, a toxic waste. Breathing also affects our state of mind. It can make us excited or calm, tense or relaxed. It can make our thinking confused or clear. What's more, in the yogic tradition, air is the primary source of prana or life force, a psycho-physio-spiritual force that permeates the universe.

Prana means energy, breath, or life force. Learning to direct and control prana in the body has long been considered a crucial aspect of yoga. As an essential bodily function, breathing is an involuntary act. Although we cannot control whether or not we breathe, we can, to some extent, control the way that we breathe. Exercises in breath control, such as breath retention and deliberate methods inhalation and exhalation for specific mental and physical benefits are at the core of pranayama practice.

The Benefits of Pranayama:

❖ Reduces the breaths needed per minute by encouraging increased lung capacity
❖ Promotes keen awareness, memory, and concentration
❖ Supports the internal organs to perform their functions with less energy output
❖ Maintains healthy blood pressure
❖ Encourages proper circulation of blood and plasma
❖ Cleans and clears the nasal passages
❖ Bolsters a healthy immune response
❖ Promotes a healthy functioning heart and cardiovascular system
❖ Delivers oxygen to the body and encourages the natural removal of toxins
❖ Supports vitality and a graceful aging process
❖ Renews all the tissues of the body
❖ Calms excess vata in the nervous system
❖ Kindles agni and promotes healthy digestion

Yoga breathing exercises are one of the best ways to lose belly fat. Known as pranayama, these exercises boost metabolism which helps to burn fats and lead to weight loss. Try these three simple breathing exercises to get rid of stubborn belly fat and regain health:

Yoga breathing can fix what expensive exercise equipment and weight-loss workouts can't. Deep breathing increases oxidation in your body leading to weight loss. The oxygen intake of the blood increases giving more energy for you to exercise. Breathing boosts metabolism which indirectly leads to weight loss. Some breathing techniques help massage your abdomen resulting in faster burning of your body fat. Now, let's have a look at some of them.

Kapalbhati Pranayama (Skull Purification)

This yoga technique is also known as the breath of fire technique.

In Kkapalbhati exhaling with all your force with the nose is important till your stomach goes deep inside. Keep in mind, only exhaling should be done completely with full force but not inhaling. Do not focus on inhaling because it will happen naturally after exhaling. Repeat this exercise for 5 minutes. In the beginning, you can practice for 15 breathing but after you can increase to 60. You can take rest for some time before starting again.

How to do Kapalbhati

Sit on the floor with folded legs or padmasana, keeping your eyes closed and your neck and back straight.Keep both your palms on your knees. Now, take a deep breath (inhale) through your both nostrils gently and exhale forcefully so that your stomach will go deep inside. As you exhale, you will feel some pressure in your abdomen. Repeat the process for at least 5 minutes.

Doing these breathing exercises regularly along with a healthy eating plan will surely give you long-term benefits.

Bhastrika Pranayama (Breath of Fire)

It is a powerful and energetic breathing exercise that raises your metabolic function and burns fat faster. Bhastrika also helps in asthma, respiratory problems, thyroid and gives calmness to the mind.

As your lungs become full of oxygen after performing Bharstika, the metabolic and other functions of the body are improved. The process of energy production in the cells is taken to the next level, as the excess of oxygen in your body accelerates cellular metabolism. Enhanced metabolism helps to remove unwanted fats and toxins.

How to do Bhastrika

Sit on the Lotus Pose with your back and neck straight, and eyes closed. Relax your stomach muscles and place your palms on your knees. Inhale deeply, filling the lungs with air. Gently exhale. Both inhalation and exhalation should take the same length of time - about 2.5 seconds to breathe in and 2.5 seconds to breathe out. Expand and contract your diaphragm in tandem with your breathing. You can repeat the procedure for 5-10 minutes.

Anulom Vilom

Anulom translates to 'with the grain' while Vilom stands for 'against the grain'. This simple breathing exercise - when performed regularly - is known to balance the Tridoshas (three doshas) in the body namely Vata, Pitta and Kapha. Most ailments are a result of an imbalance in these doshas in the body. Anulom Vilom is probably the easiest and the most effective way to stay fit and healthy.

How to do Anulom Vilom :

To do Anulom Vilom, sit in the lotus position. Close your right nostril with your right thumb and inhale gently through your left nostril. Now, close your left nostril with your index or middle finger and breathe out through your right nostril. Repeat the same, vice versa. Do this for a good 15-30 minutes.

Bhramari

The *Bhramari pranayama breathing technique* derives its name from the black Indian bee called Bhramari. *Bhramari pranayama* is effective in instantly calming down the mind. It is one of the best breathing exercises to free the mind of agitation, frustration or anxiety and get rid of anger to a great extent. A simple technique, it can be practiced anywhere - at work or home and is an instant option to de-stress yourself.

The exhalation in this pranayama resembles the typical humming sound of a bee, which explains why it is named so.

How to do Bhramari :

To do Bhramari, sit down in Vajrasana or Padmasana at a peaceful place. Your shoulders must be stretched out and your spine straight. Now, open up your palms and close your ears with your thumbs. Place your index fingers on the forehead, right above your eyebrows. Let your middle and ring fingers rest on your closed eyes. Breathe in deeply and exhale slowly, keeping your mouth closed. While breathing out, make a little humming sound.Your fingers should feel the vibrations of the sound. Remove the fingers gently from your face and rest them on your knees. One round is complete. Repeat the procedure 5-10 times.

7

YOGA MUDRAS

The word 'mudra' is a sanskrit word that is referred to as seal. The yoga mudras help seal or affirm an idea or intention. When the hand and fingers are positioned together in a pre-defined way, it generates some form of energy (prana force), which helps in healing of several ailments including overweight problems. Mudras have been in practice for ages rather since the beginning of Hindu and Buddhist traditions and it has been scientifically proven that hand mudras have various health benefits including weight loss.

They say that in mudra formation, when the hand and fingers are positioned together in a predefined way, prana force or energies are generated which help in curing various diseases and ailments along with providing weight loss solutions. The logic behind mudras is that since five elements are associated with our five fingers, practising yoga mudras or hand gestures regularly can yield several health benefits.

Finger Corresponds to Which Element

- ❖ Thumb finger – Agni (fire)
- ❖ Index finger – Vayu (air)
- ❖ Middle finger – Aakasha (sky)
- ❖ Ring finger – Prithvi (earth)
- ❖ Small finger – Jala (water)

It is believed that practicing mudras on regular basis can reap some amazing health benefits for you. Weight loss is one of them. You might be wondering how practicing mudra can help me overcome obesity. Well, for that, you need to understand how mudras work. When you practice a mudra, it activates a related body part by supplying energy to it. Once the body organs start receiving enough energy, they start performing more efficiently than before. This is how it works.

Now, for the intention of getting slimmer, you will have to perform the mudras that can stimulate the organs that affect your appetite, digestive system, and metabolism. When these three factors are stimulated, you automatically start losing weight faster than before.

Surya Mudra

As the name suggests, Surya mudra signifies the fire element and it increases the flow of the fiery energy in your body to increase the vitality and boost your metabolism and your digestive system. It also lessens the earth element inside the body which is considered to be primary element responsible for the fat accumulation inside the body. In this way, Surya Mudra helps you lean down and lose a lot of belly fat.

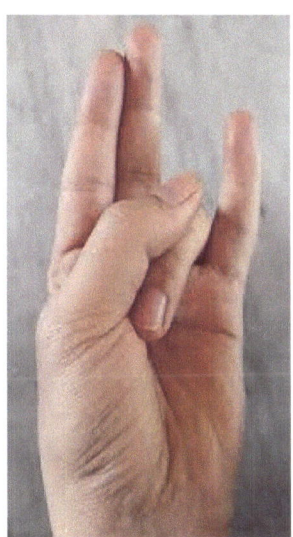

- ❖ Sit on the floor with your back straight (try to be as comfortable as you can while sitting).
- ❖ Put both of your hands on your knees with the palm facing upwards.
- ❖ Now place your thumb on the ring finger of your each hand.
- ❖ Your other fingers must be straight; only ringer finger and thumb should be bent.
- ❖ Exert the pressure on your ring finger. The more pressure you exert, the more fiery energy you will release in your body.

Gyan mudra

According to a scientific study, stress is the main reason behind over-eating and becoming overweight. Gyan Mudra is related to stress as it helps in relieving the stress from the body muscles and provides a deep sense of relaxation. This is how it eradicates the most common cause of gaining weight to help in achieving the right body weight.

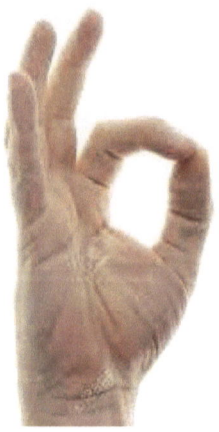

- ❖ Sit straight making 'easy pose' or 'diamond pose as you feel comfortable.
- ❖ Place your hands on your knees with the palm facing upwards.
- ❖ Cover the tip of your index finger with the help of thumb.
- ❖ Apply a little pressure on your tips of your fingers to allow energy flow through your body.
- ❖ Chant "Om" mantra for deep relaxation.

Linga mudra

This mudra is known for increasing the sexual drive in men. Just like Surya Mudra, this Mudra helps in activating the fire element in your body and thus boosting the metabolism and improving digestion.

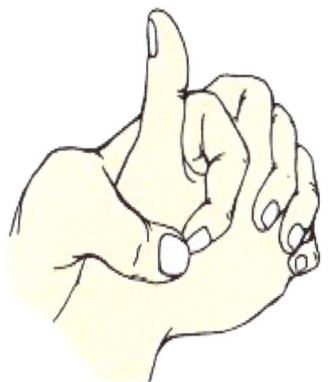

❖ Sit comfortably in half-lotus or easy position.
❖ lock your both hands except for the left thumb which must be facing upward.
❖ Place your hands on your lap exerting a little pressure on your left thumb.
❖ Close your eyes and enchant "Om" Mantra.

8

MEDITATION FOR WEIGHT LOSE

Meditation is a practice that helps to connect the mind and body to achieve a sense of calm. People have been meditating for thousands of years as a spiritual practice. Today, many people use meditation to reduce stress and become more aware of their thoughts. There are many types of meditation. Some are based on the use of specific phrases called mantras. Others focus on breathing or keeping the mind in the present moment.

Use a mantra that helps you lose weight. A mantra is a word or phrase that you repeat to yourself to focus your practice and bring you back to center when your mind wanders. As Libshtein explains, "a mantra can give you something to focus on while you meditate." Although many people find it helpful to their practice — especially since you pick something that resonates with you personally — it is absolutely not necessary. Don't feel like you need to force yourself to use one if it doesn't feel natural or helpful. If you choose to use one, Libshtein suggests repeating it to yourself as you inhale and again as you exhale. Common choices include "I am loved," "I am at peace," and "Om." If a mantra just doesn't feel right for you, Libshtein says to simply focus on your breathing.

Follow your breath to reduce stress. "Try using four counts on your inhale and eight counts on your exhale," Libshtein suggests. But meditation is all about reducing stress, so if these counts feel strained or unnatural, it's OK to deviate from them. Try to increase your counts every time you meditate. "Don't be concerned if it takes you some time to work up to eight counts," Libshtein says. "Just know that lengthening the exhale will significantly help calm you down."

All of these methods can help you develop a better understanding of yourself, including how your mind and body works. This increased awareness makes meditation a useful tool for better understanding your eating habits, which could result in weight loss.

Meditation is linked to a variety of benefits. In terms of weight loss, mindfulness meditation seems to be the most helpful. A 2017 review of existing studies found that mindfulness meditation was an effective method for losing weight and changing eating habits. Meditation won't make you lose weight overnight. But with a little practice, it can potentially have lasting effects on not only your weight, but also your thought patterns.

How can I start meditating for weight loss?

Make sure you have access to a quiet place during these 10 minutes. If you have children, you may want to squeeze it in before they wake up or after they go to bed to minimize distraction. You can even try doing it in the shower. Once you're in a quiet place, make yourself comfortable. You can sit or lie down in any position that feels easy. Start by focusing on your breath, watching your chest or stomach as it rises and falls. Feel the air as it moves in and out of your mouth or nose. Listen to the sounds the air makes. Do this for a minute or two, until you start to feel more relaxed.

1. Take a deep breath in. Hold it for several seconds.
2. Slowly exhale and repeat.
3. Breathe naturally.
4. Observe your breath as it enters your nostrils, raises your chest, or moves your belly, but don't alter it in any way.
5. Continue focusing on your breath for 5 to 10 minutes.
6. You'll find your mind wandering, which is completely normal. Just acknowledge that your mind has wandered and return your attention to your breath.
7. As you start to wrap up, reflect on how easily your mind wandered. Then, acknowledge how easy it was to bring your attention back to your breath.
8. After you clear all unwanted thoughts from your mind vizualize your body in a positive way like your body became slim and healthy, You losing fat each day etc. You can visualize you are practicing yoga too and in your mind tell that each day you are became healthy and you are lose your fat by visualization and repeating this words you will get good results.Do it regularly.

8

YOGA FOR 21 DAYS

Here I give you the 21 day time table and diet detailes.Follow this routine for 21 days.Never skip a day.....

DAY 1	DAY 2	DAY 3
Suryanamskara 1 set	Suryanamskara 2 set	Suryanamskara 3 set
Prasarita Padottanasana	Paschimottanasana	Shirsasna
Sarvangasana	Halasana	Sethu Bandhasana
Kapalbhati Pranayama	Kapalbhati Pranayama	Kapalbhati Pranayama
Surya Mudra	Surya Mudra	Surya Mudra
Meditation 5 mins	Meditation 5 mins	Meditation 5 mins

DAY 4	DAY 5	DAY 6
Suryanamskara 4 set	Suryanamskara 5 set	Suryanamskara 6 set
Vasisthasana	Dhanurasana	Shalabhasana
Pavanamukthasana	Veerabadhrasana	Bhujangasana
Bhastrika Pranayama	Bhastrika Pranayama	Bhastrika Pranayama
Linga mudra	Linga mudra	Linga mudra
Meditation 10 mins	Meditation 10 mins	Meditation 10 mins

DAY 7	DAY 8	DAY 9
Suryanamskara 7 set	Suryanamskara 8 set	Suryanamskara 9 set
Trikonasana	Dhanurasana	Shalabhasana
Pavanamukthasana	Noukasana	Bhujangasana
Bhramari Pranayama	Bhramari Pranayama	Bhramari Pranayama
Linga mudra	Linga mudra	Linga mudra
Meditation 15 mins	Meditation 15 mins	Meditation 15 mins

DAY 10	DAY 11	DAY 12
Suryanamskara 9 set	Suryanamskara 9 set	Suryanamskara 9 set
Prasarita Padottanasana	Sarvangasana	Paschimottanasana
Pavanamukthasana	Noukasana	Bhujangasana
Bhramari Pranayama	Bhramari Pranayama	Bhramari Pranayama
Linga mudra	Linga mudra	Linga mudra
Meditation 15 mins	Meditation 15 mins	Meditation 15 mins

DAY 13	DAY 14	DAY 15
Suryanamskara 9 set	Suryanamskara 9 set	Suryanamskara 9 set
Prasarita Padottanasana	Sarvangasana	Paschimottanasana
Halasana	Bhujangasana	Dhanurasana
Anulom Vilom	Anulom Vilom	Anulom Vilom
Surya Mudra	Surya Mudra	Surya Mudra
Meditation 20 mins	Meditation 20 mins	Meditation 20 mins

DAY 13	DAY 14	DAY 15
Suryanamskara 9 set	Suryanamskara 9 set	Suryanamskara 9 set
Trikonasana	Veerabadhrasana	Halasana
Halasana	Bhujangasana	Dhanurasana
Anulom Vilom	Anulom Vilom	Anulom Vilom
Gyan mudra	Gyan mudra	Gyan mudra
Meditation 25 mins	Meditation 25 mins	Meditation 25 mins

DAY 16	DAY 18	DAY 19
Suryanamskara 9 set	Suryanamskara 9 set	Suryanamskara 9 set
Halasana	Paschimottanasana	Dhanurasana
Paschimottanasana	Dhanurasana	Sarvangasana
Anulom Vilom	Anulom Vilom	Anulom Vilom
Gyan mudra	Gyan mudra	Gyan mudra
Meditation 30 mins	Meditation 30 mins	Meditation 30 mins

DAY 20	DAY 21
Suryanamskara 9 set	Suryanamskara 9 set
Halasana	Paschimottanasana
Paschimottanasana	Dhanurasana
Anulom Vilom	Anulom Vilom
Gyan mudra	Gyan mudra
Meditation 30 mins	Meditation 30 mins

DAY 21 onwards
Suryanamskara 5 set
Paschimottanasana
Halasana
Sarvangasana
Pavanamukthasana
Sarvangasana
Shirsasna
Anulom Vilom
Gyan mudra
Meditation 30 mins

Yoga Diet

In yogic and Ayurvedic philosophy, there are three qualities (gunas) of all things in nature: 1) Raja (hot, spicy, fast), 2) Tama (slow, lethargic, bland), and 3) Sattva (purity, harmony). These three qualities are present in all things, but in different amounts, making one quality dominant.

Rajasic foods are hot, bitter, dry, salty, or spicy. They overstimulate the mind and excite the passions. In contrast, **tamasic** foods are bland and include meat, alcohol, tobacco, garlic, onions, fermented foods, and overripe substances.

Sattvic food is the purest diet, the most suitable one for any serious yoga student. It nourishes the body and maintains a peaceful state. This, in turn, calms and purifies the mind, enabling it to function at its maximum potential.

A Sattvic diet will ultimately lead to true health; a peaceful mind in control of a fit body, with a balanced flow of energy between them.

If you train your body to eat at regular times, say at 10 A.M. and 6 P.M., it will better utilize its energy throughout the day as it anticipates intake of calories at these times. The body has cycles, and functions best when these cycles are regular and steady. The same goes for our meal times.

Avoiding food two hours before exercise or sleep helps the body function at its best capacity. Energy for digestion should not be taken away for the purpose of exercise. Ensuring proper time for digestion before sleep helps to keep the mind clear.

Thus, the hormones produced during sleep can be utilized efficiently to repair tissue damage and fight infection, which is ideal, instead of for digestion.

The yogis recommend choosing one day each week to fast. A fast can be strict, not allowing anything to enter the body. Or, it can include water and fruit juices. Whatever you choose, keep in mind that the goal of your fast is to purify the body and mind.

FEW LAST THOUGHTS

As a cunclusion here I giving the research article that published in www.omicsonline.org on March 26, 2013

The results of this study suggest that obese subjects who participated in yoga group show more improvement in pulmonary functions and reduce BMI compared to subjects who participated in aerobic group. This could be due to the effect of yoga postures that involves physical and mental components. This is partly in accordance with various studies, increased flexibility and relaxation. Surprisingly doing yoga it is possible to burn fat, boost the metabolism and give all other benefits to improve health. Fat burning postures explains that the backwardbending postures elevate the heart rate. Twisting postures stimulate the adrenal glands and flush out toxins.When people think of yoga, they think of its wonderful benefits like mind and body connection, increased flexibility and relaxation. When doing yoga it gives the quick effect on body. That will get one's heart into its target zone. Yoga can help to develop long strong muscles a flat stomach and a strong back along with improvement of posture .Of course, these physical changes are depends on other lifestyle factors, such as a well-balanced diet and regular physical activity. Most of the studies have shown significant weight loss by regular yoga practice. One study found that after three months, healthy adults lost an average of 6kgs. For weight loss program, all obese participants reached and sustained a normal weight with continued practice of yoga within one year & showed improvement in pulmonary function [8].

Regular aerobic exercise and strength training are productive, but aren't the complete answer. Yoga may be just the piece, need to complete the puzzle of keeping both the body and the mind fit. Yoga exercises are performed with very few, but extremely precise, repetitions in several planes of motion. In yoga, one focuses on breathing, and therein lies its healing. Breathing itself has extraordinary healing capacity on physical and emotional levels. Current research indicates pranayama the conscious breathing is more helpful to improve pulmonary function

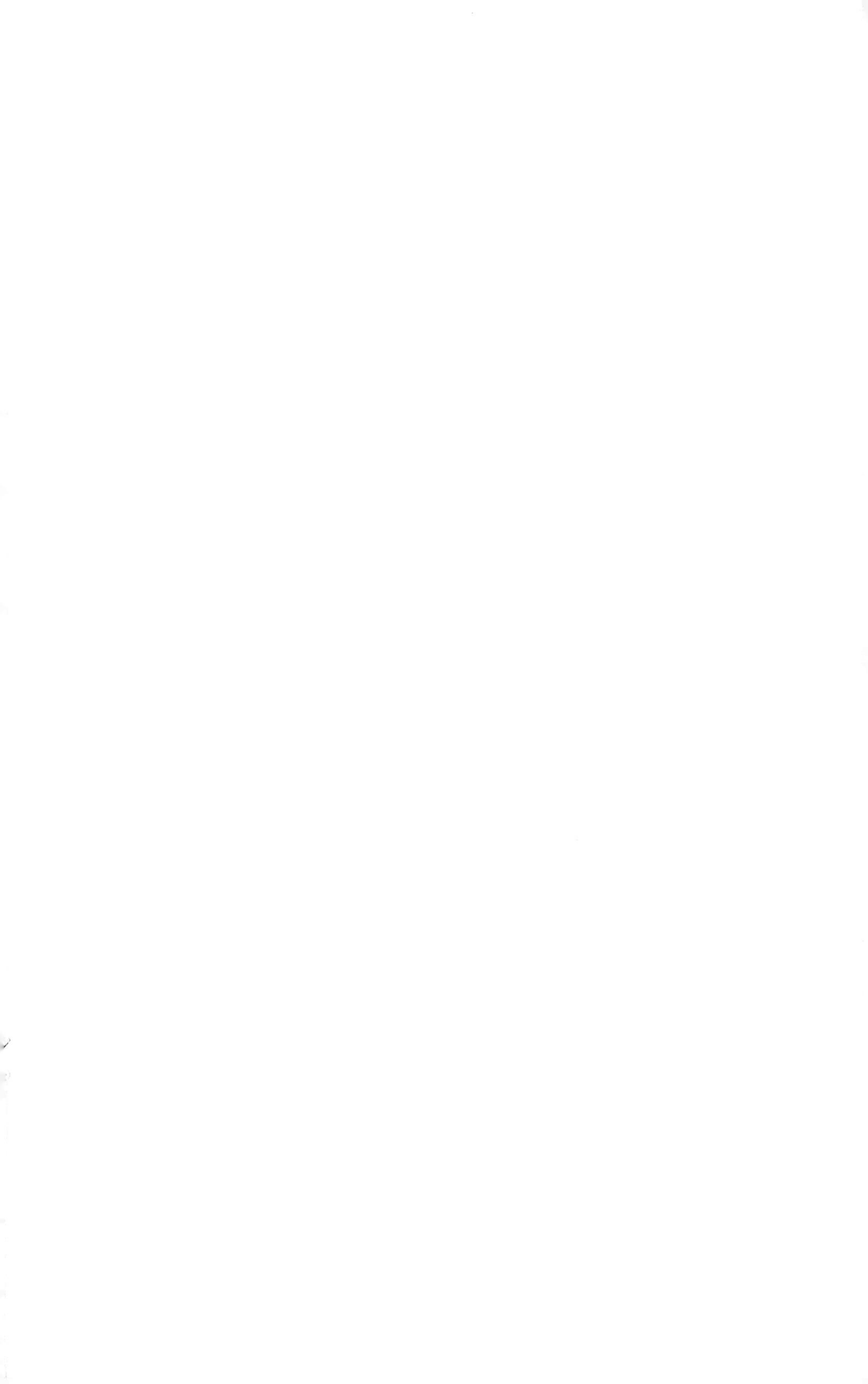